LIVE FOREVER:
THE SHOC DIET

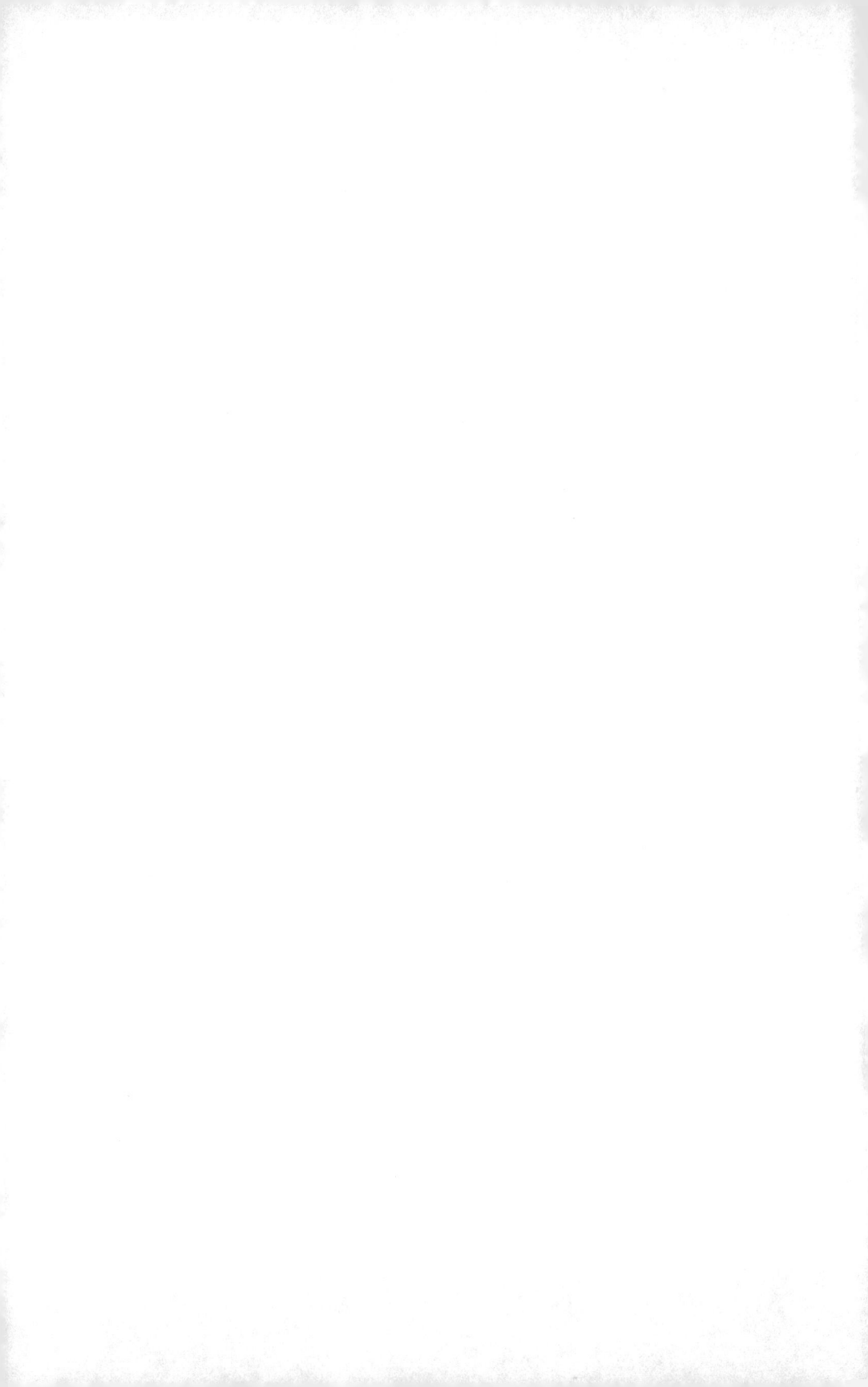

LIVE FOREVER: THE SHOC DIET

Buy this book!
This is the most important book you will ever read

Dr. Harris Michael

To order additional copies of this book, contact:
Xlibris Corporation
1-888-795-4274
www.Xlibris.com
Orders@Xlibris.com
38200

Buy this book; it could very well save your life!
The little book that could help you live forever . . . read on friend
Introducing the "SHOC" diet.

As with any health or diet book it is important that you check with your physician before undertaking any change in your diet or exercise routine. Please discuss with him or her the changes you want to make and your plans. The recommendations here can help you but you need to tailor it to your particular situation.

The SHOC diet

1   time for you in the morning

     A learn pray meditate/learn something every day 1 hour defeat disease/psyllium and 'bulk' it down
     B Yoga, motivation,
     C exercise routine

Aerobic and weights ; positive thinking/wear step meter

2   diet

     a protein is your friend; count calories and your weight
     six meals
     and let's design them now

       bfast:
          oatmeal/banana
          special k
          eggs

       snacks:
          bars; peanuts; fruit

supper:
>   fish/chicken/lamb
>   salad

dessert:
>   orange; apple' healthy choice ice cream/smart start

lunch:
>   shake to eat
>   soy
>   oatmeal
>   walnuts

3   vitamins from a to z

1   a,b,c,d,e,flax, folate, lutein, lycopene, magnesium, asa
2   salmon and fish oils
3   daily weights and charting your progress
4   goal setting and daily routine for this
5   off day; party time
6   Thanksgiving and that family touch
7   tests for your heart a ct, mri, crp, lp(a), homocysteine
8   defeat anxiety and worry

>   a   act as if and then act to help
>   b   so what; be solid

9   can't change your family
    juicing daily/flax
    slimfast
    frozen dinner
    liquid
    strawberries

CHAPTER 1

The SHOC diet stands *for 1 strenuous exercise 2 healthy eating 3 observing biometric data 4 contemplation.* This diet and way off life was born out of the need I had to help my patients. Today more than 2/3 of the people ever to live over the age of 65 are alive.

We need to find a way to not only live longer but to live healthier lives. In my experience I have seen many people that have a diagnosis of heart disease or cancer. Many of these are young people.

Many forms of heart disease can lead to heart failure or stroke. You can imagine the concern people go through when they are given this diagnosis. The usual thoughts of 'why me' and what will the future hold comes to mind. Only after time and the thoughtful approach of their doctors do patients come to grips with their condition and gain a new acceptance and perspective on life. I have seen this time and time again in my patients. Many young people come in diagnosed with a serious illness and they break down. Only after time and an awareness do they come to a realization that the control they once felt was actually artificial. They realize that our lives are transient and that at any time our lives could change. This book is designed for you in a four step program to take control of your health and your emotional and spiritual existence. These are intertwined. Studies have shown that people that have good coping techniques for stress suffer less from cardiac problems including sudden death. What will follow in the remaining chapters is a sort of blueprint, sometimes with exact ideas and recipes with you can live till probably one hundred years and live those years in full control of your faculties and in a healthful fashion. We will explore issues of weight and weight loss as well as look at some measures of your cardiovascular health that should be addressed. With the advances in technologies that are available there are many people that need not die prematurely. The process of technology is evolving and I hope through this journey together that I can make this more understandable for you.

The precept of the diet and contained in its name is the idea that you will vary your routine every 60-90 days. This will "Shock" your body but also through the components in the acronym it will allow you to live a full life and eliminate what I believe is an entirely controllable disease: coronary artery diseae.

We will discuss many vitamins and options available to you for living to your potential.

Finally a detailed study of meditation and yoga will be discussed. Our minds and bodies often function as one. It is important that we realize this and allow for full synchronicity of our "Chi". We have three faces, what the world sees, what we see and the way we really are. When we are not in alignment with these three we have stress and dysfunction manifests itself as illness, depression, anxiety and worry. We need to align our life force and being. I will offer you some techniques and ways of thinking that will help you in your day to day life. Stress comes from people and from money. Whether they are the people at your workplace or at home and if you are concerned about money you are in the majority. We will examine ways that you can deal with all these issue.

CHAPTER 2

Strenuous exercise

The value of regular exercise cannot be overestimated. Medical study after study has looked at this issue. People that exercise live longer and live better. The issue of the type of exercise and duration is somewhat debatable but you must do something. You will hear what my bias is in terms of this and I will try to provide you with some rationale for this. You will need to exercise to lose weight and to stay healthy. Please contact your physician before undertaking any program.

You probably have heard that you should exercise three times a week. I fell you should everyday! For 20 minutes to 1 hour it is necessary. I am a morning person and prefer to exercise in the morning. You can do it in the evening if you are so inclined. Some people say that if you exercise in the morning you burn more calories during the day. This may or may not be true. The bottom line is you should do some. The program that I recommend for optimal cardiac conditioning and weightloss is weights with some aerobics on three days and full cardiovascular on the other three days. For the one day a week that you rest, you should do extra meditaition, yoga and tai-Chi.

For your weights the first day will be arms and this will be the triceps and biceps. Usually you should do two exercises for the triceps and three for the biceps. Using free weights is fine or even if you use a universal this is acceptable. After one set of ten reps I recommend increasing your heart rate by vigourous cardiovascular such as doing the stairmaster or treadmill. Do this just for a minute or two then go back to lifting the weights. If you choose to workout in the morning you should start the day with about a half hour of meditation. This can include prayer if you are a religious person. We will speak more of meditation under the "C" of SHOC.

Definitely don't listen to the news when you first get up. It is discouraging usually and you should wait till later in the day. The first hour is critical for the day. If you are a student you should listen to some tapes during your workout and if not you should choose something that you can learn from your work or something motivational. Anthony Robbins has some wonderful tapes and really has a wonderful system. There are a lot of other motivational speakers and tapes and I would encourage you to find someone that is uplifting. This is a great way to start the day.

Make sure you design your goals as far as your weights. The body mass index should be your height divided by your weight. This should be below 25. Obesity is abundant in the United States and is a cause of tremendous morbidity and mortality.

CHAPTER 3

This is a diet and living book. It is a book that will help you with your health and living. It is born out of years of medical study and practice. There are many things that doctors can do to improve your health but there are also things you can do to help yourself.

What I will attempt to do is to give you the tools to live a long long life but also life that life in a state of health that means you have a quality of life. This book is not expensive; what I would like in return from you is not a lot but it is something. I would like you to commit those extra years you will live to meaning something and I want you to start now.

Whether it is volunteering at your child's school or making an effort to give away used clothes you owe me this. I would like you to do something good for someone else; in some sense to "pay it forward" and pass it on. Please do this. You will live much longer and better if you follow my book and teachings and all I ask of you is that you make it mean something.

So many of my patients really don't have a good quality of life and can't get very much out of their existence. The first thing I will tell you is that you need to take a half to one hour in the morning to meditate and do yoga and plan your day. Later on in the book you learn specific techniques that can help you with meditating and with those you can dramatically reduce your stress level and your cholesterol values.

To start in the morning get up, let your feet swing off the bed. This will let the blood reach your feet. Then get up and have two glasses of water. This will wake you up and hydrate you.

Consult your doctor before starting an exercise program. Next you should do some yoga. Online there are some great poses. I particularly like downward dog as well as sitting down and outstretching your feet.

Yoga has been around for many years and is a great way to stay in shape and stay young. I would suggest you buy some dvd's on it. Another great form of exercise and relaxation is Tai Chi.

In fact there is data to show that seniors that do tai chi in fact have an 80% less risk of falling. The slow motion and stretching along with the deep breathing helps the lymphatic system and keeping your blood pressure low.

So if you start your day with proper hydration and stretching like yoga you are off to a good start.

Tony Robbins is a great motivational speaker. He on his "personal power" program advises you to read positive material and to start the day with positive questions like "How did I get so lucky?"

Also take the time to plan your day as to what you are going to accomplish.

It is a good idea to list your priorities in terms of what you want to do that day. In fact you should have it listed for the week as well. When you prioritize it is important to work on the most important items. That way when you accomplish something you are then able to strike off the most important thing. If you have five things to do and only accomplish the first three you are still making progress.

The morning is also a good time to take your vitamins, more on that and your psyllium and fiber. An important part of the "live forever" philosophy is to have healthy stools.

What I mean by that is to have a large volume of stools. The less time that a meal has to sit your body the less time it has to give off carcinogens and fatty components and acids. There are actually some studies that show the healthiest people have the largest volume of stools. You actually can improve this with eating more bran and whole bran cereals.

The morning is a good time to just do five or ten minutes of a walking meditation.

Now it is time for you to get into your exercise routine. In the morning is the best time to exercise as you don't need to sit and evaluate whether you will do anything. It should be as routine and natural as rolling out of bed. You should alternate aerobic and anaerobic training. For weights you can do circuit training or just plain old weight lifting with taking breaks between the sets.

I would recommend exercising in the morning so your heart rate will be elevated all day.

For the aerobic part if you exercise for thirty minutes three times per week that should be fine. For the weight lifting part if you do it two to three times per week you should be alright. There are different types of weight lifting but I recommend doing chest and back on one day and then arms and legs on another day. At first you can choose to do heavier weights and lower reps. Ideally I would like you to be able to do 4-6 sets at 10-12 reps

There are various routines you can use. Right now I have started something called "Escalating Density Training" where you have a fixed amount of time and you try to increase the number of reps you are able to do. Once you are able to increase them by about twenty percent you then go ahead and increase the amount of weight you are lifting. Rodale books has a great book on this. My point is that you need to vary your training and for weights every say two months you probably should take a week off from them. Your body tends to get used to a particular routine. Circuit training where you mix in some aerobic activity is actually very good as well. There is even a school of thought that says you should do four minutes of high intensity aerobics then for four minutes do lighter weights. After being on call or when I don't have a lot of time I will do the escalating density routine for fifteen minutes. It depends, but I will tell you that you need to keep developing changes in your routine. I would recommend a main sport or learning a new one. I started back at golf this year and it helps in terms of focusing your goals but anytime you do something new with your body you are decreasing the chances of developing Alzheimer's disease.

We are not training to be body builders here and you really want to prevent the onset of osteoporosis. Your workout is important. I would recommend changing it every couple of months. For example if you are running for a couple of months maybe you could switch to the treadmill after that. Your body gets used to a type of stress and what this does is create a different type. This is part of the cycle of life. We need to continuously challenge our bodies. By taking the time we need in the morning we set ourselves up for the rest of the day. I would recommend swimming for one or two days out of the week. It is a great exercise and for most of us as we age we need something that will not be hard on our joints at all. This is a terrific exercise and works all major muscle groups. Also you can run in place or do karate kicks in the water. You can pretend you are lifting weights or doing lunges. You can also do a water yoga routine. This is really a wonderful medium. You should incorporate water training into your routine. It will also help chronic low back pain.

I particularly enjoy listening to classical music. This definitely decreases your stress response and physiologically helps you to lower your blood pressure and heart rate.

It has been well documented for children if they listen to classical music they will 'get smarter'. The idea is that the mathematical patterns help with organizing the brain and helps us understand order better. A study from the University of California found it was more relaxing than listening to jazz or silence. I recommend listening to classical music for a half our a day. You can do it while you are working out or in your car.

You definitely need a satellite radio system. It is well worth the 12.95$ per month. You are able to listen to whatever music you want. Music has a powerful effect on our memories and often our favourite songs "bring our minds back to a happier time".

For example first thing in the morning I will listen to a half hour of a motivational cd like Carleton Sheets or the Time Quotient system just to get psyched up. After this I will turn on the Sirius TM and listen to the 80's. I grew up in that time and have fond memories of all the songs. So when I listen to "Celebration" with Kool and the Gang I am really back in Junior High on a basketball on the road trip. I will talk a little more in the meditation section about controlling your thoughts and creating pleasant thoughts.

There is new research from Dr. Abraham Kocheril in Champaign Illinois looking at the value of harp music. Apparently listening to it can help regulate your heart rate after heart surgery. About thirty percent of people will have their heart go 'out of rhythm' with the surgery and listening to music is supposed to help.

So in summary in the morning it is very important for you to stretch, be grateful and do some exercise. It is also a great time for you to go ahead and plan your day. Lanny Basham is a world champion shooter. I highly recommend his tapes. He talks about 'mental management'. It is a wonderful program that focuses on the mind.

It teaches us to focus on the one event and to picture it in our mind. So, in the morning if for example you are an ad executive you could picture yourself having a meeting with your big clients that day. You picture your lunch break and coming home. As a physician I started doing this and even though my day appears hectic it actually is very smooth as I have already thought of most things in the day. While I am on the topic of thinking of the day I do recommend physically writing out your day plan for the day before. The key is to look at this the day before. Writing things out helps you immensely. We will talk about this later but I would recommend for example you everynight and morning writing out your weight goals. For example I write, I weigh 165 lbs. Now, I weighed this when I was in the eight grade and now weigh 169lbs. This is pretty good. I am fourty years old and have the same weight I did when I was thirteen.

My point is, is that I picked a goal that is reasonable. I wasn't content with the goal of 170 or 169 but chose one that is reasonable and reachable. When writing your goals it is important that you look at the five dimensions of your life. They are 1 your spirituality 2 your health 3 your family 4 your job 5 your finances and future achievements in terms of career. I actually have a digital recorder that I keep in my car and used it to act as affirmations for me. I will record myself saying "I am a hard worker or I have a good temperament and I control my anger". Also I have ones that say "I weigh 165 lbs". Now by writing and saying these things out loud you are sending the message to your subconscious mind that this is the goal.

For your plans for the day when you make it up I would like you to use a file card system and write down only the most important things first. So you can put down your meetings and things that need to be done. When you get them done you can cross of a particular item. By focusing on the higher number items you will tend to get the important things done. Steven Covey talks about the important and non urgent and that is where you want to spend your time. So at the end of the day even if you didn't get everything done you were able to at least get the most important things done.

So every morning you should be excited to start the day and tackle your list of things to do. Also, meditation is a great way to get centered.

While on the topic of satellite radio and controlling the input to your mind and body I would highly recommend getting Tivo TM or some variant of it. You can program what you are going to watch and you don't need to bother at all with commercials if you don't want to. When you come home from work or even if you are home during the day you can control everything that is put into your mind from the tv.

Some people say it is a 'wasteland' but frankly I think it is a wonderful tool for knowledge, entertainment and relaxation. I particularly enjoy watching CNBC for businesss news. There is a show by "Cramer" that is just fantastic. It really is a great way to learn in a fun way about the stock market. As far as comedy goes there is a terrific show based on a British comedy called "The Office". This is a great show. Also on Comedy Central there are a lot of very funny shows. I would recommend at least ten minutes of a comedy as this has been shown to be like an aerobic workout.

This chapter had a lot of information in it. Each point is very important and I want you to think in detail about it. In future chapters we will go into detail on the SHOC diet as well as nutritional supplements and vitamins.

2   diet
    a protein is your friend; count calories and your weight

    six meals and let's design them now

    bfast:
         oatmeal/banana
         special k
         eggs

    snacks:
         bars; peanuts; fruit

    supper:
         fish/chicken/lamb salad

    dessert:
         orange; apple' healthy choice ice cream/smart start

    lunch:
         shake to eat
         soy
         oatmeal
         walnuts

This is just a basic outline of the diet. In the morning you can be a little liberal on the carbs. I try to have you not eat any carbs after about 12 noon. If you do eat them they are very limited.

This diet is sort of a mix of the high protein diets as well as the Mediterranean diet which is really the only diet that has been proven to lower your cholesterol as well as some cholesterol medications. We will talk a little more about plant sterols as well. These can lower your cholesterol about 25%. If you combine them with a statin, which is a class of drugs very potent at lowering your cholesterol you will be very successful at reaching your cholesterol goals. In the morning I do recommend orange juice and a red juice. By a red juice I mean grape juice or pomegranate juice or the latest juice in North America, Xango juice. This is a juice that is from the Mangosteen in the far east. These juices are very high in anti-oxidants. Oxidation is a process that is key to inflammation; most major illnesses are related to inflammation. If you can control inflammation you can control cancer, heart disease and a variety of other chronic ailments like diabetes and arthritis. Also this is a good time to have some fruit.

After working out you can manufacture another healthy meal. In all you should have about six meals a day. The snack meals in the middle of the day can be a piece of fruit like an apple or a healthy protein nut bar. You can have water with it. I recommend 6-8 glasses of water a day.

For snacks throughout the day you can eat nuts, fruits, apricots, apples or oranges. You get the idea. I don't want to constrain you so much you don't have the choice of what food you want to eat. You know what is healthy. On the other hand I want to give you some idea about what to eat.

For lunch I recommend a salad, a liquid lunch like slim fast or a protein shake. By switching to a liquid diet you can easily drop a lot of weight quickly. Then at around 3 pm I recommend another snack.

The dinner should be a fish like wild Alaskan salmon or tilapia. I would recommend it a couple of times per week. Fish oil tablets or Carlson inspected fish oil are also very good. You want one that is inspected so you don't have to worry about the mercury content. The other issue of course is the pcb's. These can cause cancer.

Other dinners can include white meat like chicken or turkey. If you must eat beef you can eat lean cuts and only once a week or couple of weeks. I recommend eating all food well done.

You can eat hummus with pita bread and garlic. The garlic pills are fantastic as they are packed with nutrients and are able to lower your cholesterol and blood pressure.

At night a glass of mild with cinnamon or almonds is also nice. You can have a light snack like a weight watchers tm dessert or the like. I recommend going for at least a ten minute walk after eating as this dramatically increases your digestion. This will help you before you go to sleep.

You should not eat three hours before sleeping. This will allow your digestive system to work properly. I would also recommend some fiber supplement like psyllium. Another option is fiber supplementation like benefiber tm. One school of thought maintains that the larger your stool volume the longer you will live!

I think it is important that you get to a point where the food doesn't spend a lot of time in transit. What is nice is when you eat the food passes through you. By moving quickly through your body there is less time for the food especially the acids to stay and cause damage. Many foods like meat are actually carcinogens, meaning they cause cancer, so if you can have the food stay for only a little time in the stomach you will be allright in terms of the meat not having any affect on you.

If you can try to eat a salad for lunch or even a liquid lunch like a slimfast I think you will be on the right track. Always be thinking what your last meal was and what the next one will be. Walnuts, peanuts and almonds are great sources of protein and great snacks. The nice thing about protein is that it is an appetite suppressant and it doesn't ad a lot of fat to your body. It helps your mind mainting it's sharpness and goes right to muscle building. The AHA diet was off when they kept pushing refined sugars.

Oatmeal is a great breakfast or anytime meal. Something I like is power oatmeal is putting some almonds and nuts and apricots on the oatmeal. Then let it sit with a cover over it for about fifteen minutes. Add some brown sugar and honey and this will keep you going for the day. It is terrific at lowering your cholesterol as well. You can crush some flax seeds and add them as well. For men I advise staying away from flaxseed oil as this has been linked to metastatic prostate cancer.

Soy is something that is a great source of protein for women. For men again I would advice taking it in moderation as it has been associated with estrogen like effects. This isn't ideal . . . also it seems not to be that beneficial in terms of men's minds. There is plenty of nutrition out there without putting yourself at risk.

So to summarize, you are to eat six meals a day with snacks included. Portions should be small, about the size of your fist. That is one reason that frozen dinners are so good for people trying to lose weight. You cook them in the microwave then you put them on your plate. By doing this you are using a smaller portion so your stomach shrinks and your body gets used to this.

You will get one day where you can eat any three meals you want . . . yes you heard me right! I encourage people to do this as it is easy to stick with a diet when you know every seven days you will get to eat whatever you want. Also with a strict diet your body gets used to 'starvation' mode . . . this way you are teaching your body that there is plenty of good food and keeps you on your toes. I would encourage you to look up the Mediterranean diet on the internet as well as the South Beach diet. You can vary your routine a little, but by sticking to healthy food that overall restricts your calorie intake you should do fine. Common sense in moderation is the major piece of this plan. Eating right should be simple, you should be able to accomplish your goals with the plan I outlined. Experiment and try things like nutrisystem™ and weight watchers™. The key is that you cut out the fries and fast food hamburgers and the full desserts. When you want to eat ice cream make sure it is low carb and low in fat. This is common sense. As they say though, common sense is not always common practice!

CHAPTER 4

Vitamins: let's talk . . .

What I wanted to do in this chaper is to address the many issues surrounding vitamins and herbs. There are a lot of good things out there.

Let's jump right in and start with vitamin a. This is a something that you need to be careful about if you are pregnant. This is a terrific vitamin for your eye health. This should be part of your multivitamin complex. Another thing for eye health is lutein. There is good evidence this can help in terms of macular degeneration.

Vitamin B is essential as a stress vitamin and there is data to suggest that is does lower your homocysteine level. Homocysteine elevation is thought to be related to vascular disease. I would encourage you to take a b complex along with folate. Also if you take biotin every couple of days this will help your ability to concentrate and focus. Bee pollen greatly helps in terms of arthritis and joint pain.

On this topic I recommend vit e with fish oil and a 'red juice' like grape juice or pomegranate juice. This combination will act as an anti-inflammatory agent.

This is just as good as taking an asa or Tylenol. There is something about the vit e antioxidant affect and the fish oil that is really very beneficial.

Of course as Linus Pauling has been telling us for years the use of vitamin c as an antioxidant is well known. I recommend 1000 mg daily.

You can divide it up into two times per day. It is very useful in keeping your mind and body active.

Vitamin D is helpful for bone density but it also helps to decrease hypertension.

Lycopene is particularly beneficial in preventing cancer. It can be taken separtately or can be present in tomato juice or sauce. For example, pizza will contain this.

Fish and fish oils as we talked about are very important in keeping triglycerides down as well as preventing heart disease.

Magnesium helps to stabilize the heart rhythm as well as calcium. It also is very good at lowering blood pressure. If it seems like a lot to take all these pills I recommend taking some in the morning and some at night. The fish oil, magnesium and potassium are best taken at night. Most heart attacks occur in the early hours of the morning.

Aspirin should also be taken at night; it has more of an effect on the blood pressure if this is done. This is a great drug. If you are a man over fourty or a woman over fifty you definitely should take it. It is just as good as a lot of the 'clot buster' medicine used for heart attacks. It's anti-inflammatory properties are very good at decreasing an important marker of heart disease called the crp level.

We will talk more about this later.

We talked a little about garlic earlier but there are many spices and herbs that are beneficial. Specifically there is an Indian spice called mehti that really works to decrease blood pressure. You take the mehti and ground it down. Then you wash it and dry it in the oven for about fifteen minutes. It is then in a powder form that you can mix with a drink or water. It has been effective for centuries. Another good remedy for coronary disease or more so for prevention is bilberry extract. You can buy this at the drug store and it is effective at preventing atherosclerosis or hardening of the arteries. Cinnamon in the form of powder or pill is very effective in regulating sugars. Diabetes and inflammation are a key component of coronary disease. I recommend you take it at night so sugars will be regulated through the night.

L-arginine is one of the new players on the scene. It tends to increase the nitric oxide which is important at preventing the oxidative effects of stress. I would encourage you taking this daily or every couple of days.

Turmeric has been used for centuries in India to prevent cancer. An Indian physician friend of mine told me how stomach and colon cancer is almost unheard of in the Indian subcontinent. For people with heart problems they often prescribe almonds. I recommend eating a good Indian curry meal once a week and if you can't do that there are turmeric tablets you can take every couple of days. These treatments like garlic are well known across many cultures as being beneficial for health. They must work if Ukranians, Chinese and Indians use the same thing. They are from different areas of the world and they came up with the same conclusions. There are many medications and herbs like this that are 'cross cultural'.

Coenzyme Q is a great supplement to take especially if you are taking a statin. This class of cholesterol lowering drugs actually can deplete the supply of coenzyme Q which is worrisome. It is a drug that is useful in regulating the heart rate as well.

Plant sterols or 'phytosterols' are a great way to lower your cholesterol almost 25 %! They can be as beneficial as some classes of the statin drugs. You can go to the website "Heart Guardian™" to buy this or go to Wallmart and buy "Nature's Made Cholest-off™". These are great products and natural ways to lower your cholesterol.

L-Lysine is also a great supplement to take to increase your nitric oxide in your body and cut down on the oxidative stress. L-arginine also increases the nitric oxide.

These are all terrific ways to help your body work naturally to prevent and fight disease.

In fact mentally you can do a lot to fight disease. Say, you played and enjoyed football. If you have leukemia with a decreasing white blood cell count you can imagine that the white blood cells are the enemy quarterback and you are linebacker just lining up and tackling him. Or, if you play ping pong you can imagine you are defeating in ping pong the breast cancer that you have. This won't take the place of chemotherapy obviously however the exercise will help in terms of fighting the disease.

To summarize I recommend taking these vitamins and supplements twice a day in divided doses. You can also work on the first half of the alphabet and the next half the next day.

Vitamin c, multivitamins, garlic and potassium and magnesium should be taken daily. Check with your doctor especially if you have any kidney failure as potassium and magnesium may not be the best thing for you.

CHAPTER 5

Daily weights and charting your progress

I read a book on weightlifting by Schwarzenegger and he said you should weigh yourself weekly. I on the other hand think you should weigh yourself daily. By doing this you will be able to see if you are making real progress of if you are falling behind. If for example you notice your weight is up then you need to cut back on your meals and maybe just drink liquid meals that day. You may need to cut down on salt and increase your water production. Charting is very important.

I recommend it for your exercise routine as well as for how much weight you lift. It is an important part of your progress. How can you lift more if you don't know how much you already lift? How can you walk further if you don't know how far you normally walk?

I would encourage you to weigh yourself daily and to keep track of whatever progress you can make in terms of your weight and activity.

It is important for you to check your heart rate and blood pressure on a regular basis. This will help you keep track of your progress.

CHAPTER 6

Off time is very important for your body and mind. The time you take off with your mind helps it relax and convince it that you have plenty of time left.

Downtime or building some margin your life is so important. I tell people that you should have one day where you eat whatever you want. That is a twenty four hour period that you can eat cherry pie and Big Mac's and not feel guilty. It is one of the best ways you can keep on a diet. Otherwise it can be very difficult. If you give yourself something to look forward to it will be a lot a easier for you. Also for your workouts you will need to take a day off. Then every 6-8 weeks you will need to vary your routine. This applies to both your aerobic routine and weight lifting routine. This is very important because it sort of "Shocs" your body to enable it to adapt to a the new stresses you put on it.

Also during your regular activities it is important for you that you don't schedule things too tightly. I will tell you if you if I have patients to see at 9 am I try to get there around 8 or 8:30 and I relax, eat breakfast, joke around with staff and casually examine the charts of the patients I am going to see. So many of my colleagues will try to cram their morning rounds in before and will arrive late for their patients. I would rather 'add' a little time at the end of the day to get the work done. What I'm saying is you will actually get more done if you build some room in. I will actually just take a week at half speed to get caught up, not because I think I 'need' it but because 'a change is as good as rest'. We need to pace ourselves. I used to think that I wanted to 'retire' early and have all this time off. I actually one year took three weeks off in a row and I tell I you it was a little boring.

This gets to the next issue. You will need to take at least twenty minutes in the morning and the evening to meditate. Studies have shown that people that meditate live longer, have less heart attacks and are more at peace than people that don't.

There are many different forms that this takes. One is the TM method where you repeat a phrase or 'mantra'. This was made very popular in the 1960's and is still very popular. Doing this focuses your mind by repeating the same words. Meditating is to me like happiness. I don't just say "I'm Happy" . . . . I do in affirmations but truly I do something at work or at home with my family and I say "Gee that made me pretty happy." It is almost by letting go and not searching for it I am able to get it. I use the term "I" in the hope that this will generalize to you. It probably will. With meditation you can feel anxious and wound up but for you to make the trip to the 'other side' and be relaxed with everything you need to let your mind relax. Then when you are done with your session you are like "Hey I feel pretty good and calmed down. Try taking your blood pressure before and you meditate and you will find it goes down quit a bit. If you have some vacation or some time off force yourself to up your meditation time to 1 hour or more a day. There is a Buddhist saying that "When you are have time you should meditate for a half hour; when you don't you should meditate for an hour!" This is very true.

Another meditation method is where you are simply aware of the different body parts. For example you close your eyes and concentrate on your right hand then each finger. You feel it getting hot then getting cold; then you feel the wind on it, then fire then water. You then move on to each finger then your wrist then your arm then you go down your body. When you are meditating you then breath and say out loud whatever you focus on. For example if you notice your breath you just say "breath" or your stomach then you say "stomach". Another variation is where all you think off is your breath as you breath in and out.

Something I like to do is if I think of something I like and I picture it in a picture frame of my mind; if it is a noise I listen just to that. The point is by doing this you occupy your mind and clean it out.

The paradox is here: the less 'clutter' and anxiety you have in your head the more you will have. You will be more productive; wealthier and better socially.

I started doing this and my professional productivity went up several fold.

The gratefulness meditation is where you just think about everything that you are grateful for. This is a wonderful way for you to start the day.

Another meditation technique is to just count ; yes just start counting. Sometimes I start and can't get past like three! Why? Because if you are counting you need to restart if another thought enters your mind! This is a terrific way to 'unclutter' your mind and one of my favourites.

Another basic meditation method is when you think about pleasant memories; past or future. By doing this the endorphins get released as you relive or experience this. Why do people have their radios stuck on the "Big 80's"?

Was it because the music is so great? Yes it is but it is also because it takes us back in our minds to a simpler time; a time when we were happy, secure, carefree. Yes this is a very powerful method of controlling your mind and physiology. My blood pressure has dropped 20-25 points after just a simple meditation session. It is amazing. You cannot escape the 'trap' of daily life and its' routines. What I'm telling you to do is to try to create these "oasis" points where you can carry yourself through the day. Often people turn to alcohol, drugs, sex to fill these empty places but by living properly you can fill these voids in a healthy manner.

Another thing I encourage people to do is hypnosis. There are a variety of tapes and cd's that can help with this.

I will say you need to clear any addiction before you can move ahead in your soul and mind. This is simply by showing restraint.

I tell my patients that smoke that I know they smoke because they enjoy it and it feels good. I don't agree that telling kids that 'drugs are bad' or that 'you feel aweful' works. I think we need to say 'yes, drugs make you feel good . . . for now' but you shouldn't do them because first off it is wrong. This message seems to be missing from all the commercials. Simply making a moral judgement is missing from our society.

It is wrong for teachers to have sex with students; it is wrong to drink and drive. Period. We shouldn' t have to tell people they will go to jail. People are weak and don't want to show restraint. So many of my patients are obese. Eating makes them feel good; but in the end it is not good for them. The first step in beating the addiction is to say "I know this is pleasurable in the short term but it is not right!" It is that simple. Whether the person is addiction to alcohol, food, drugs, gambling, sex . . . it is all then same.

Now I will give you a simple way to beat any addiction. You need to subsititute one addiction for another. So when you get the urge to have a cigarette you go ahead and walk or 'pace' and do this for ten minutes. Then you will meditate or "ponder" and you do this for also ten minutes. You don't think or try to rationalize. You then call a friend that will support your. This is similar to the AA sponsor issue. Finally taking a shower, cold, will cause your mind to be distracted. This should eliminate any desire you have for food or alcohol. You need to respond to your craving constructively.

We are often too "non-judgemental" in society. I will tell you that drinking too much, smoking and lying and committing adultery are all bad things. Some in society are talking about "traditionalists" well; this is traditional. If you live properly and stick to these values you will live longer and feel better. I didn't say that your goal was to 'enjoy' your life or to be 'happy'. What I said was you would live longer and in the end feel better. So many patients I have that are in their 90's when I ask them what is their secret they say "clean living". Now if this is your goal then read on and implement what I tell you. If you are like some of my patients that are fourty five and drink to excess and smoke and don't care about their own lives or the lives of their families then this book and it's recommendations are not for you. You don't care about others and I have news for you; the rest of us don't care for you. The self destructive losers out there can stay in their own camp. This book is for good people that are trying to live a long and productive life. I'm not saying we are all perfect; I am saying that by aligning your values and living properly you can not only respect yourself when you look in the mirror; you have a high likelihood of living a long and healthy life. No, I'm not trying to judge you but I am encouraging you to judge yourself and do so honestly.

Some very basic things that you can do involve smiling about a dozen times for like a minute every morning. Simply by doing this you will feel better and studies have shown that you will in fact look younger; yes this is a side benefit of this. Smiling makes you happy. I saw an add for a popular steak place last night and it said 'Leave your problems behind; life will still be there in the morning!". That is a major principle that we are talking about. I'm not talking about walking around every second of every day 'ecstatic'. I'm talking about restoring balance to your life. This morning I'm going to play basketball with my friends; I know that when I get paid I'm still going to have to deal with lawyers in a malpractice suit that is baseless; that my father will still be sick and that I will have the same problems someone else like me has. I say this because you could say "oh you make like close to a million dollars a year what problems do you have?".

Believe me I have friends that are very very wealthy through medicine, business, oil, farming and the like and I have friends that are not wealthy and all people have some sort of problem. As long as we walk the earth we will have problems!

Think of that as a natural truth just like "the world isn't fair". You can like or dislike it but it is a fact. The good guys don't always win and people don't always get what they deserve or what you think they deserve! That's the way it is in real life ; not in a Hollywood movie!

Having said all that there is karma and we will be responsible for what we do.

So every day in addition to trying to learn something new I would encourage you to do at least one good deed. This could be small like opening the door for an elderly person or giving someone a rose or helping someone that is lost.

This will make you feel good and it will help your 'karma'. Also try to say "hello" to a stranger or give them a genuine nice greeting. Don't be one of those people that are so caught up in their own lives that they can't see anything beyond this.

The luckiest and most successful people will greet you and talk to you and make 'small talk'. People that can't see outside their own existence and problems are small and petty people; don't be that way. See the big picture and try to be magnanimous. That is why websites that link people are so successful. We are stuck in our own world but can't connect to our fellow human being which we crave so much.

By now you have probably figured out if you do the things I tell you to the byproduct will be happiness. Yes you will be happy with yourself, your family and your friends. It is ironic; that if we sit and ask 'are we happy' we probably will not get there and this is a waste. If we find meaning in our lives by what we do and how we act ultimately I am sure you will be happy. I am middle aged and if I died tomorrow I would be satisfied I dedicated my life to helping others. I am not happy because I got drunk or committed excesses that would 'make me happy' I have an inner satisfaction that my life was lived properly and I helped others. This satisfaction produces inner strength and yes happiness. Strive for this and you can do this through meditation and contemplation.

Doing for others will help you sleep better at night and will bring happiness.

It is strange but by focusing on others outside your own sphere you through a combination of distraction, compassion and gratefulness you will achieve a level of happiness.

There is evidence if you meditate you will lower your blood pressure, look younger and have less cardiac events. Try not to work weekends; there is evidence this increases your stress. Also, there was a study that showed people that were not refreshed after a weekend had a much higher chance of a heart attack. In fact this was increased by three times.

CHAPTER 7

Thanksgiving and that family touch . . .

It is important to keep contacts with your family and social contacts. This is very important. However there is a little dilemma on how to see your family without wanting to jump off a bridge . . . . yes . . . they can drive you crazy. There is a fine line. When people that emigrated from Italy to Pennsylvania but kept their same lifestyle in terms of having family around, walking everywhere instead of driving and really not changing their diets actually lived much longer than the many other Italians that immigrated to the US. A lesson there is how important social contact is. This has become much easier with the internet available. You can email and send instant messages and send pictures. I would encourage you to meet one new person a day; simply greeting them counts. Also I would ask that you try to send an email everyday. That means you can send it to one of your classmates or someone from your past. This method of keeping in contact with people will help you.

By maintaining close social contacts you will feel connected. As human beings we all have this need. It is important for us to see our families. They love us and have seen us over time. They know us. Whatever materialistic or career goals you may have there is no subsitite for good friends or a strong social network.

Brian Mulroney the former Canadian Prime Minister used to send Christmas Cards to everyone he met or was vaguely acquainted with. What was one thing he was well known for? His 'network' of friends and contacts of course! Everyone is so busy and caught up in their own lives that you will really stand out if you are someone that can take time to talk with people and actually connect.

As our society drifts further into an isolationism ie home entertainment, ipods, icasts, tivo . . . if you can actually connect with someone it becomes that much more meaningful. This is a demonstration of a principle in business called a 'network effect'. The more people that you connect with the more valuable each connection becomes. You feel like you are intertwined in this network of existence. This serves as a method of support for you but also builds on your sense of meaning and existence. This connection is what we all want and now it is much easier to achieve.

Your family is your original beginning. They knew you "back when". Keeping this connection sometimes is hard. You definitely need to visit your parents on holidays if possible; that is a few times per year. This will cement the bond you have. Now with the internet you can take pictures and send emails and instant messaging. By doing these things you keep contact. When my wife is away we try to talk, send emails and I send flowers whenever I can. As human beings we need to keep in contact. This fluidity is important in any relationship.

With your relationships you will have a very immediate or 'circle of trust' in terms of friends but also you will have some looser friends then some more then acquaintances. What I am saying is try to keep some contact with everyone to some degree. I still play chess with my high school physics teacher and we haven't seen each other in close to twenty two years. It keeps a sense of connectedness and purpose and meaning. We don't live and die alone. We are social creatures. My parents have a shzit shu dog and when we are all at the table he just wants to sit with us. He just wants to be around us. This isn't because he wants anything;

just to be part of it. Humans are the same way. This is a way that we can avoid depression and loneliness; a big problem in today's society. Computers and technology in the 1970's they said was going to make our lives easier. Well I don't know about you but I don't seem to have a lot more time! No simply having computers is not the answer; the answer is being connected to one another. This idea of wireless and connectivity is where it is at.

Try to understand that this is an important part of our existence and you need to let it breath.

Your family can be a touchstone; forget the slights and perceived offences of the past. There is something called the "Sedona" method where you just let things go.

This can help you tremendously. If you just let things go and and try to realize you need to move forward. Sure you could be mad at your mother and father over certain things in your childhood or how they treated the other siblings compared to you but you need to go ahead and try to get over it. "Move Along" like the song says! By sitting down and planning family get togethers you will find that it adds meaning to your life and keeps you connected. I'm not talking about living on the same street but I am talking about keeping in contact. You need the family touch just like you need a network of a few friends that you can trust and communicate with.

Study after study has shown people that maintain some connection with a social network will live longer. They also will live better. Make no mistake, I want you to live a long time but I want you to make a difference in the time you spend on this earth. This translates to living well and helping people and making a positive impact while you are here.

CHAPTER 8

Tests for your Heart

In this chapter I would like to review with you some of the different tests that are available for your heart.

The main thing we want to make sure is that you don't have a significant build up of plaque in the arteries. Now this plaque starts to develop at a very early age.

Just having a 'blockage' doesn't mean you will have a heart attack. If you look at pregnant women who smoke you can see their fetuses already have developed blockages in the arteries or 'arteriosclerosis' as we call it. In fact, in 19 year old men there is the development of the disease. In prostate cancer we say people die with the disease and not from it. This is partly true with heart disease. In fact, most of the disease can be treated with aggressive medical treatment. There is a belief and a want on the part of people to think that in fact if they just have heart surgery or just have an angioplasty, placing a balloon or stent into the artery that they will be all better. This really isn't the case. Because simply progression of the disease is not what causes the heart attack. The 90% blockage doesn't just progress to a complete blockage. What is much more likely is for a 50% blockage to rupture and cause a heart attack. Generally with balloons and stents we treat 70% blockages or above. An exception to this is the main heart artery called 'the left mainstem' where the two main branch arteries the lad and cx originate. In fact once this gets to 50% we tend to treat it.

So it seems we might be 'stenting' or treating the wrong arteries.

So, keeping this in mind we need to see how we can decrease our risk for heart disease. It is the number one killer of all diseases.

I recommend knowing your numbers. What I mean by that is checking and recording your blood pressure and heart rate at least two times per day. Also it is important that you have your cholesterol checked. In terms of the cholesterol I recommend knowing the total cholesterol, the ldl and hdl and triglycerides.

There are some other more in depth markers but these are the ones every single person should know and keep track off. They have some great products on the internet where you can even check your cholesterol with a home kit.

Your ldl ideally should be below 60 to really prevent and cause a regression of heart disease. The triglycerides should be less than 150 and the hdl should be greater than 55 for men and 65 for women. The hdl as many of you know is the so called 'good cholesterol' and it is effective in 'mopping up' the bad cholesterol or ldl. Ldl stands for low density lipoprotein.

There are new methods for looking at the heart. Something like a 64 slice ct scanner is useful in creating a non invasive way of looking at the heart arteries. This is not 100% accurate but carries much less risk than an invasive or traditional angiogram where doctors thread a catheter through your groin up into your heart. If this heart catheterization carried with it no risk we would do it on anyone and everyone. Because of the cost and risk we don't; the degree of radiation is similar to a heart cath. You might have heard of a cardiac mri; that is not something that we do to look at the heart arteries. It is mainly looking at the heart muscle and looking for evidence of a heart attack. It is essential that you have some sort of marker for disease. A C reactive protein tells you about inflammation and your risk of potentially having a heart attack. Lp(a) is also a newer marker of heart disease as is homocysteine. Although recently homocysteine has not been shown to be helpful in terms of lowering it lowering the risk of heart disease. I would recommend you definitely have your cholesterol checked and probably do so annually.

If you are over the age of 40 or have a family history of heart disease I recommend some sort of stress test or a ct angiogram of the heart. Every single person needs to have this done so we can catch early those people with significant coronary artery disease and those at risk for having a cardiac event.

This is very important.

Go to your family doctor and say you want a stress test and or to see a cardiologist. Depending on your particular situation in terms of where you live and your insurance and the nature of your doctor's practice this will vary.

What I am trying to encourage you to do is to be aware of your cardiac situation and to try to take steps to make yourself better if you can. Maintaining a proper diet and regular exercise help but you need to know what your risk is.

The main point of this chapter is to understand what your risk is and manage it.

The worst position you can be in is to be at risk and not know it.

CHAPTER 9

Deafeat Anxiety and Worry

People are stressed over their family, money or job. This is the majority of people. I have seen so many people in my practice and I can tell you that this is definitely the case.

The first thing we will tackle is how to defeat your anxiety or fear of the future. The fear is something with an exact cause or something that you are concerned about ie losing your job, your spouse. Anxiety is a generalized fear without anything specific. What I would tell you is try to imagine the worst case scenario and work backwords. What if you lost your job? Would the world end? No it would keep going with or without you. So you need to see what you would do.

Well in the short term you would probably panic as you wouldn't know how to pay your bills and you would be embarrassed in front of your friends.

Then in the end you would find something. The fact of the matter is that the employment rate is about 95% in this part of the world. Would your 'friends' treat you differently? Well maybe but then they aren't your real friends are they?

The other thing is just to try to do something to protect you should the worst case scenario actually occur. For example if you are worried about losing your job you could take courses for another career so you would have something to fall back on if you did lose your job. By going through the worst case scenario you teach your mind that you can handle anything and you don't worry. I don't advise thinking of this too too often as this will cripple you with fear and anxiety. It will give you confidence to know you can deal with things.

CHAPTER 10

Restrain yourself please!

This chapter in contrast to the messages of "search" for your bliss; be happy; "are you happy yet?" will approach life from a different standpoint and premise. We will suppose that our only purpose is simply not to be happy but rather to live a disciplined and principled life no matter how long it is. Of course a long life is what we are all striving for but the question is "why are we doing that?" We need to ask ourselves if our life has meaning and everyday are we living in a way that strengthens and is in line with the vision of ourselves and our life?

I will ask you to show restraint. That is show it when it comes to smoking, drinking, alcohol and other vices. You may not be entirely successful in stopping smoking but you are making the effort and that is really what counts.

More people are overweight than are hungry in this world. We are facing new challenges in that we need to show restraint.

We are overweight because we enjoy eating. We like doing that. Also for people that use alcohol and drugs it is the same way. It is not like, these things make you feel bad. We need to be honest with ourselves and our kids and the fact is yes, initially there is an immediate benefit to these things. We need to focus on the long term pain. For alcholol for example look at its relationship to domestic violence, car accidents, driving while intoxicated. These are the things that happen when we go for the immediate pleasure of life. We need to use our heads when we decide to have that extra drink or consider smoking. We need to just lay down the law on our kids and say "Yes this maybe pleasurable but don't do it because it is wrong!". This is a message that is sadly missing. The same is true for gaining weight. We need to realize the short term pleasure isn't worth the long term pain of overeating.

I'm going to teach you a technique that can stop any behaviour. First say you wanted to stop smoking; I would advise you to buy many of the cd's out there that deal with hypnosis to stop. Listen to the cd for an hour during the day. That is listen for a half hour in the morning and half hour at night.

Then when you get a craving you should do this; 1 take a cold shower; this will take your mind off smoking. 2 You should walk for at least 10 minutes and do push ups and sit ups to distract your mind 3 you need to meditate as I have taught you for 10-15 minutes and finally you need to call a friend 4 for support. This is similar to the techniques in the Alcoholics Anonymous. Also what I would like you to do is to pay yourself ten dollars for every day you avoid alcohol and buy something nice with it. However, if you fall back you take whatever money is accumulated and give it to charity! This works for kicking any habit like drinking, doing drugs or smoking or even overeating. Another thing you can do when you are meditating is think what your life will really be like in 1 year, 3 years and 5 years then 10 years if you keep this up. For example you could picture yourself with lung cancer and never seeing your grandkids grow up. You could visit a hospital wing or a cancer center to reinforce this pain. To substitute whenever you want a cigarrette you should look at a picture of your grandchild and know that is why you are staying healthy. Each time you go to the fridge to overeat keep a picture of you as obese or as fit as possible to guide yourself with 'pain and pleasure'.

This method of stopping harmful behaviours will work for you as long as you know the 'why'. For example, you could say you want to stop drinking because you don't want liver cirrhosis or you don't want to kill a child as a drunk driver.

There are a lot of reasons. You need to stay slim so you can avoid diseases like hypertension, cancer and heart disease. Think about the life you have and how it could all end in a second with a health problem. This is not just any health problem but one that could actually be prevented. That is sad.

We will then talk about how you deal with tragedy when it does occur to you as it inevitably will.

The whole idea of a lot of books is to suggest how to 'be happy' and 'be fulfilled'.

I would submit that it is more important to do the right thing and follow the rules.

If you do that then you will not go wrong. So many problems exist because we cannot control our own desires. Whether this is related to the 'beast' of being angry or in the form of addictions it is simply a lack of restraint. I saw an episode of a popular televsion show saying that marriage was the way to happiness and not sleeping around. The same is true of the drug commercials; we all remember the 'this is your brain on drugs'. The problem with that is that it is not true to a lot of people. Many young people do drugs or know people that did drugs or their parents did. They are not 'fried'. In the 1950's we used to say not to do these things because they were wrong. That should be all there is. It shouldn't be that if you are not happy it is wrong or if you get pain it is wrong. I knew a lot of doctors and still know a lot of doctors that sleep around and get pleasure from it.

I believe this is wrong. Sure you put yourself and others at risk for disease but simply saying something is wrong should be enough for you to stop it.

For example, with eating properly and living longer. You should do this because it is the right thing to do. There is nothing wrong with telling your kids not to watch a particular show or to avoid drugs. These things are wrong.

When it comes to your health and living a proper life I have tried to outline some of the things you can do to live a longer and more meaningful life. I've been blessed to spend my life as a physician and helping others. I'm not asking you to do that. If you work a job at a factory, take pride in your work and try to volunteer say on Saturday for little league or try to donate your time to fund raising.

It doesn't matter what your religious belief is. Nothing will make you feel more satisfied and rewarded then spending your life helping other people. If you are depressed or feeling in a low mood by helping someone else not only will you forget your own problems but you will feel good about yourself. I will tell you a secret; by living a proper life defined by right and wrong and by helping someone else you will in the end be very happy and fulfilled. It is ironic that through the open search for happiness and gratification we often cannot achieve what we seek; by forgetting ourselves and living properly we will gain the meaning and bliss we all are looking for.

In this book I have given you many tools for living a longer and more meaningful life. I would like to make the case for living right. Also, please as repayment to me I would like you to do something good and live with a noble purpose in action, deed and thought. The life you have is a gift; how you live it is your gift back.

Remember, you can live your life as an example or as a warning; be an example of the wonderful potential of the human spirit. Be good and live long!

http://www.shocdiet.com/

www.ingramcontent.com/pod-product-compliance
Lightning Source LLC
Chambersburg PA
CBHW021931170526
45157CB00005B/2275